FAQ TEEN LIFE™

FREQUENTLY ASKED QUESTIONS ABOUT

Athletes and Eating Disorders

Barbara A. Zahensky

ROSEN PUBLISHING
New York

Published in 2009 by The Rosen Publishing Group, Inc.
29 East 21st Street, New York, NY 10010

First Edition

Library of Congress Cataloging-in-Publication Data

Zahensky, Barbara A.
Frequently asked questions about athletes and eating disorders / Barbara A. Zahensky. — 1st ed.
p.cm.—(FAQ: Teen Life)
ISBN-13: 978-1-4042-1807-9 (library binding)
1. Eating disorders in adolescence. 2. Athletes—Nutrition.
I. Title.
RJ506.E18Z34 2009
618.92'852600835—dc22

2007051057

Manufactured in the United States of America

Contents

Chapter one

WHOSE BODY IS IT?

Do you or anyone you know want to become an athlete but feel that eating too much will affect your athletic skills and performance? Do you diet constantly, take diet pills, or occasionally eat lots of food in a short period of time (called bingeing) and then purge the food that you just ate by self-induced vomiting, taking laxatives, or giving yourself enemas? Are you obsessed with becoming too heavy or with exercising and practicing for many hours each day? Are you uncomfortable with your body? Do you compare yourself with others in your sport or on your team and think that you need to be thinner to be competitive? After all, it is your body, and don't you have to look a certain way to perform well in your sport? If you change your eating habits or your enjoyment of food, will you improve your performance on the team?

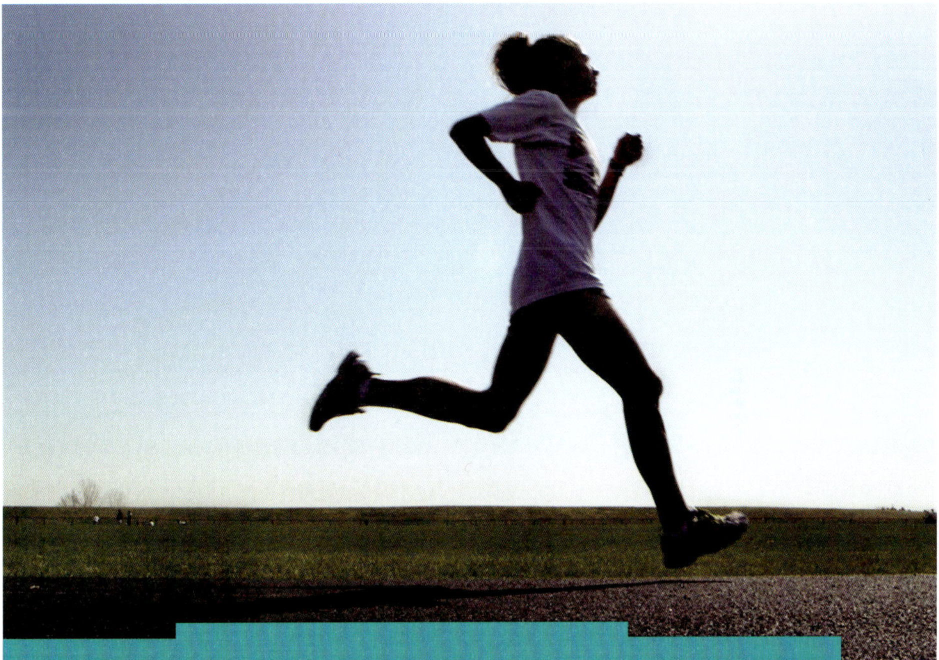

Many athletes exercise excessively to achieve their ideal weight. However, overexercising and undereating can have negative health effects.

If you or some of your friends have these thoughts or feelings, you aren't alone. Researchers estimate that as many as ten million females and one million males in the United States have eating disorders. The prevalence of eating disorders among athletes resembles that of the general American population. One 1999 study found that out of 1,445 college athletes, 9 percent of the female athletes needed treatment for an eating disorder and another 58 percent were at high risk for developing disordered eating behaviors. For males in the same study, 1 percent had eating disorders and 38 percent were at high risk for developing eating disorders.

Many teen athletes, anxious and unsure about the relationship between food, weight, and performance, make unhealthy eating choices. Too often, these athletes have extremely limited diets and weight-loss "secrets," which become patterns of deprivation that they cannot stop without help. The eating disorders anorexia nervosa and bulimia nervosa are the most extreme examples of these patterns. Anorexia is an eating behavior that is characterized as self-starvation. Bulimia is a repeated cycle of overeating, called bingeing, and then getting the food out of the body before it can be digested, called purging. These disorders are not fads, bad habits, or ways of expressing personality. Anorexia and bulimia are categorized by health professionals as psychiatric illnesses that require medical and psychiatric or behavioral treatments until the body recovers and the symptoms go away. The pressures of competition in sports; the social emphasis in the media on being thin; and family, peer, or personal problems can put athletes at risk for developing eating disorders.

Many young athletes, including some outstanding performers, have ended their sports careers and hurt their bodies with severe dieting, fasting, purging, and other measures. Often, they do this in the hope of improving their performance or impressing others. In recent years, the news media have reported the deaths of a nationally ranked female gymnast, a young ballet company member, and a college wrestler from illnesses and injuries that began with disordered approaches to food and exercise. Many

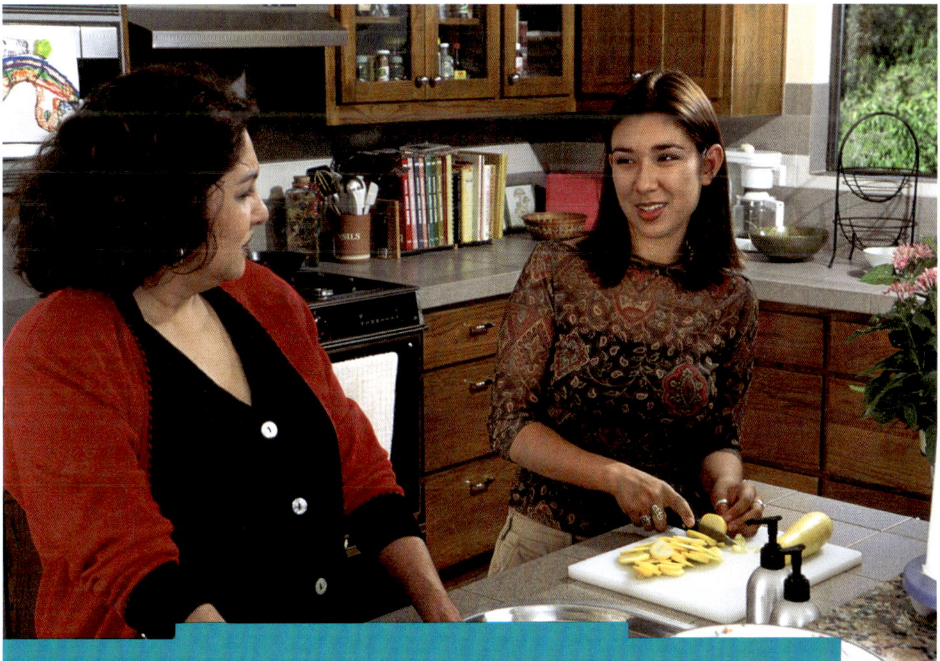

It's always wise to talk to an adult or a nutrition expert if you feel that you may be developing an eating disorder.

other less famous people have also lost their lives to eating disorders. Most medical researchers agree that among mental illnesses, eating disorders have the highest death rate. Furthermore, the mortality rate of anorexia nervosa is twelve times higher than for all other causes of death for females between the ages of fifteen and twenty-four.

If you think you might have an eating disorder or know someone who does, learn about what eating disorders are and why people with disorders need help. It is not a substitute for treatment, which doctors and psychologists provide. You can educate yourself, though, to prepare for discussions about food and health with a friend, family member, or trusted adult. But do not try to treat yourself or anyone else you think has an eating disorder.

Whatever your reason for wanting to know more about athletes and eating disorders, reading about eating behaviors will give you information to make decisions and find support to help you play hard and live well.

The "Right" Type of Body

Athletes and performers are not the only people who can feel anxious about whether their bodies are the "right" type. Teenagers, especially females, watch themselves very closely and worry that they're being watched and judged all the time. Unfortunately, there are real reasons to feel as if people are watching. Sometimes it seems as if everybody, from disk jockeys to the males at school, has something to say about the "right" kind of female body and face.

Commercials, magazine articles, music videos, and billboards focus on women's bodies. Television cameras zoom in while sports announcers scrutinize every play and player. In some sports, even the uniforms and hairdos are rated! And instructors' or coaches' ideas about the "right" kind of body for dancing, swimming, diving, cheerleading, or basketball can be almost impossible to ignore. After all, aren't they the experts? With all these messages, it's hard to remember that other people's opinions are not the only determining factor in your success or happiness.

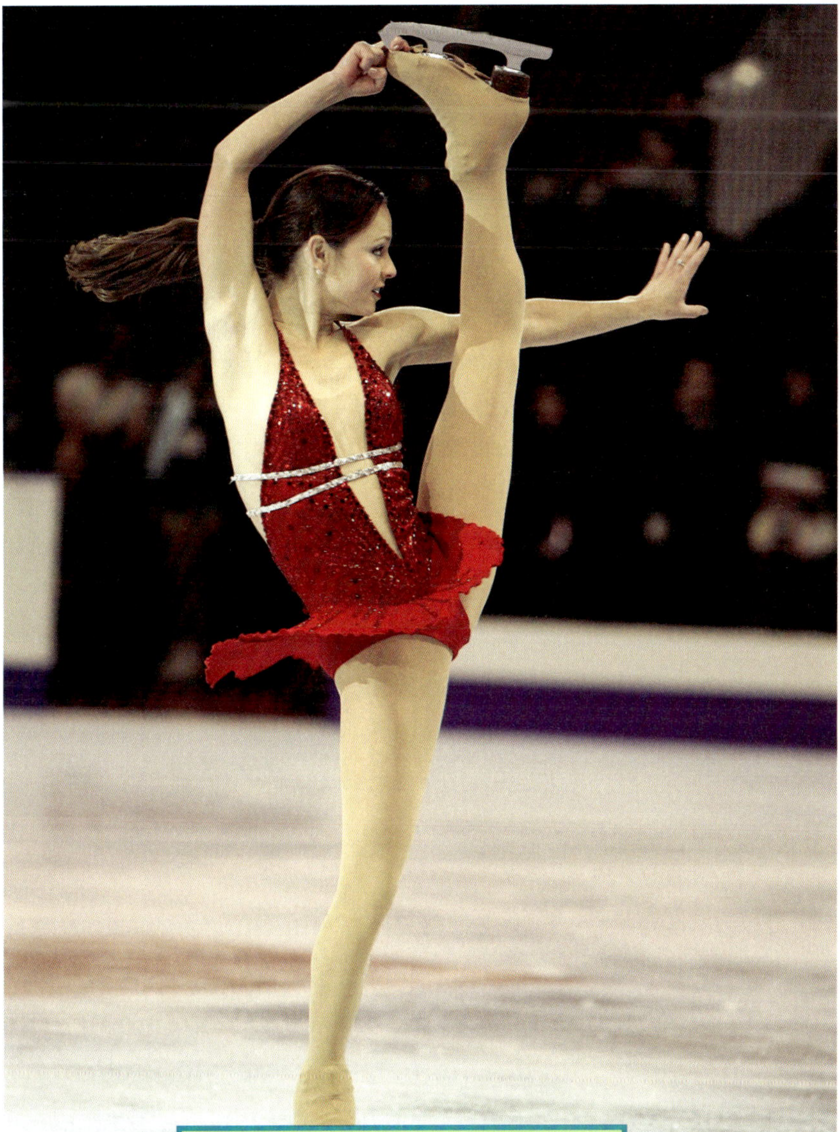

Endlessly striving for perfection often drives many athletes to develop eating disorders with the hope of performing better at their sport.

In sports such as track and swimming, the clock picks the winners. These athletes work on improving their speed. The only question is: Who finished fastest? In team sports, points are awarded for getting a ball through a net, goal, or fence that are the same for all players. They work on their scoring and defense skills. But gymnasts and figure skaters win competitions with votes from the judges. It's easy to see how an athlete competing for the judges' favor can focus his or her training on copying the body or the diet of a top-ranked star.

Some fans admire sports stars for their "victory" over food or fat as much as for their skills and style. When skaters are praised for following the same sugar-free diet for several years, or football players are admired for eating twenty hot dogs in one sitting, their athletic ability is connected to their eating habits. This connection makes self-starvation or binge-purge cycles seem almost typical for many athletes.

Who's on Your Team?

Many coaches and trainers give advice about nutrition and meal planning to student athletes, especially in major sports like wrestling and football. Other coaches may not have the time or knowledge to give their athletes more than vague encouragement to "keep up your strength" and "do what you have to do to feel your best."

Students who aren't taught how to follow a training or high-performance diet may experiment with unhealthy habits. They may pick up bits of nutrition advice from infomercials, older students, and magazines. Or they may simply try to achieve the

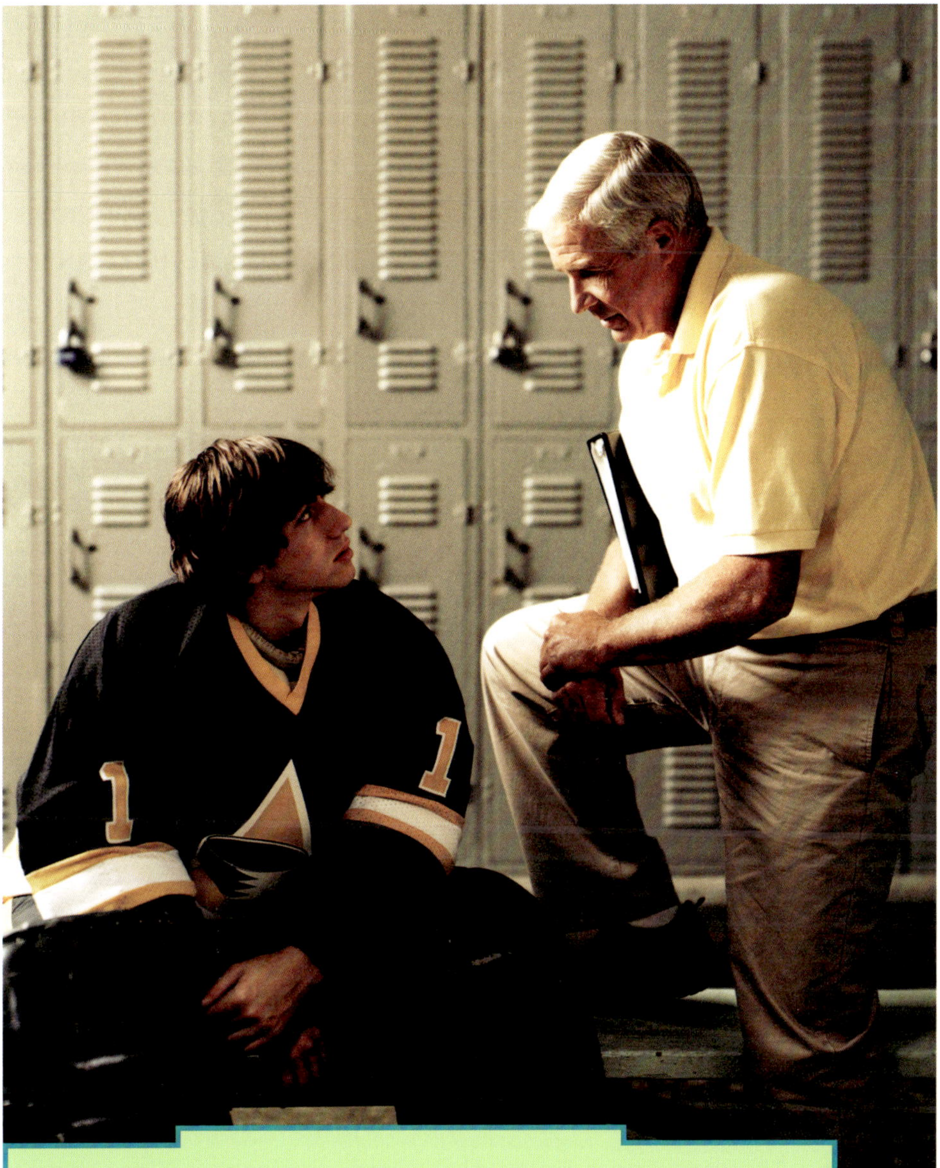

Though you should listen to your coach about training and diet, it's also important to listen to your body if you feel that you're not getting the nutrition you need.

things their coaches praise most—competitive intensity, desire, or perfectionism—by taking one or two food guidelines to hurtful extremes. A gymnast whose coach tells her to "lighten up on the pasta," for example, might respond by cutting many other carbohydrates out of her diet and eating only fruits and vegetables. (There are gymnasts who are vegetarians. Ask your doctor, nutritionist, school nurse, coach, or guidance counselor about nutritional vegetarian diets for athletes or where you can obtain guidelines for balanced vegetarian meals.)

A coach can have a winning record, superior knowledge of the sport's rules and strategies, and great motivating skills, yet he or she might not know a lot about "eating to win." In most states a person does not need to take a nutrition class to become a physical education teacher or a coach. (However, many coaches and trainers do have up-to-date knowledge about nutrition, and many schools teach nutrition in health classes.) One survey of exercise instructors found that most of them had wrong information about the power of food and exercise to change a person's body. Just as important, a coach may not recognize that an athlete is losing weight because of an eating disorder.

Pleasing Your Coach

Disordered eating or exercising may begin as an effort to please a coach. Athletes may willingly, even secretly, follow harsh self-imposed rules. In Michigan, a college wrestler died after working out for hours in a rubber suit that kept his overheated, dehydrated body from cooling off. According to teammates, he

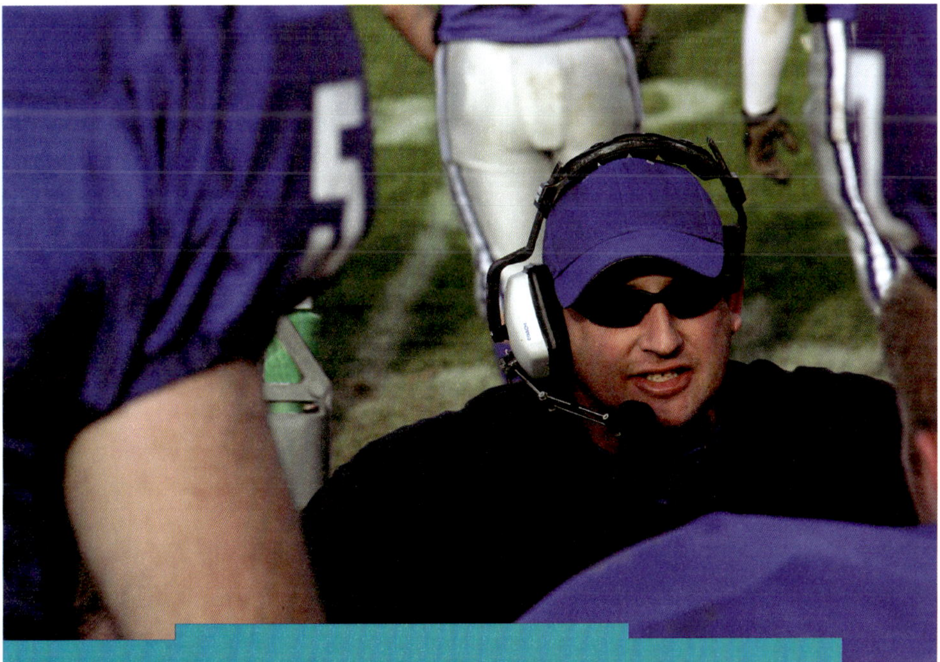

Coaches and teammates demand your best performance, but it's important not to sacrifice your health to achieve such goals.

was attempting to "sweat out" and "burn off" 12 pounds (5.4 kilograms) in one day to make his weight.

Lisa Ervin was a teenage figure skater who moved away from her parents to live near her coach and prepare for Olympic competition. *Inside Edge*, a book about competitive figure skating, tells about an episode during Lisa's training when she gained a few pounds and her spins and jumps became a little weaker. When her coach pointed this out, Lisa volunteered for weekly weigh-ins, secretly fasting before each one and bingeing afterward.

She also punished herself for poor practice sessions with long workouts on an exercise bike. Lisa did not develop a full-blown eating disorder, but many young athletes who begin similar routines for quick weight loss soon have an unbreakable habit and an eating disorder.

Coaches can put extreme pressure on athletes to perform at the highest levels in a sport. To make this high level, athletes have to have a competitive edge in their sport. So, to keep going at a high level or to improve to an even higher standard, athletes will find ways to be better. If athletes have the mentality and personality to be superior—perfectionism, compulsiveness, and expectations of high achievement—they will think nothing of putting their own well-being and health at risk if that means it will improve their athletic performance.

Chapter two

HOW DOES THE BODY PROCESS FOOD?

You were born with a unique genetic heritage. You have a mix of biological traits that were inherited from your mother and father and built into all your cells. When babies grow into girls and boys and then women and men, why do so many people suddenly expect their bodies to have a "right" size and shape unrelated to family traits? Doesn't it make sense that your bone structure and metabolic rate (the speed at which your body uses food for energy) are influenced by genetics, as much as the curl of your hair and the color of your eyes? Genetics matters more than diet, exercise, or any other single factor in determining the shape and size of people's bodies. It does make sense, and medical research has confirmed that it's true. Scientists who studied a group of adopted babies throughout their lives found that in size and weight, they were more like

Though diet plays a great role in your weight and strength, genetics may be an even more influential determinant.

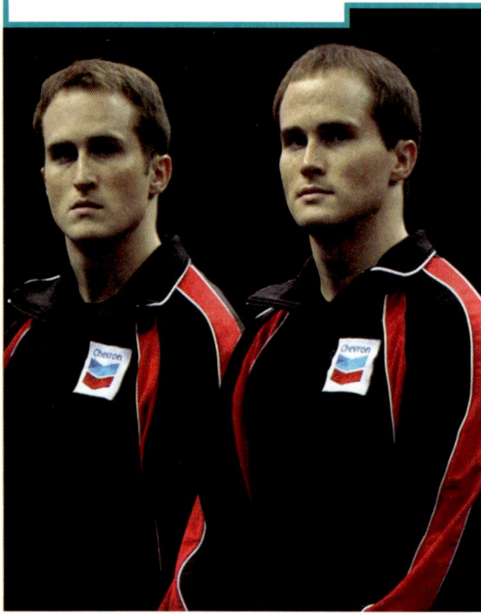

their birth parents than their adoptive parents. Similar results were found for sets of identical twins who were separated and raised in different families. With nothing in common except their genes, they grew up with virtually identical weights and body builds. So it's not entirely true that "you are what you eat."

All Bodies Need Fuel

If you're an athlete, should you eat like one? Do you need more or different foods than less active people? If you practice and train, you are exercising. You need to eat more calories than if you weren't working out. When you exercise, you use up more energy. Your body does need more fuel than less active people.

In fact, you need calories for much more than just your workout. All the things you don't even think about doing require more energy than a one-hour practice. That's because your body's "work" is going on constantly, renewing and replacing your

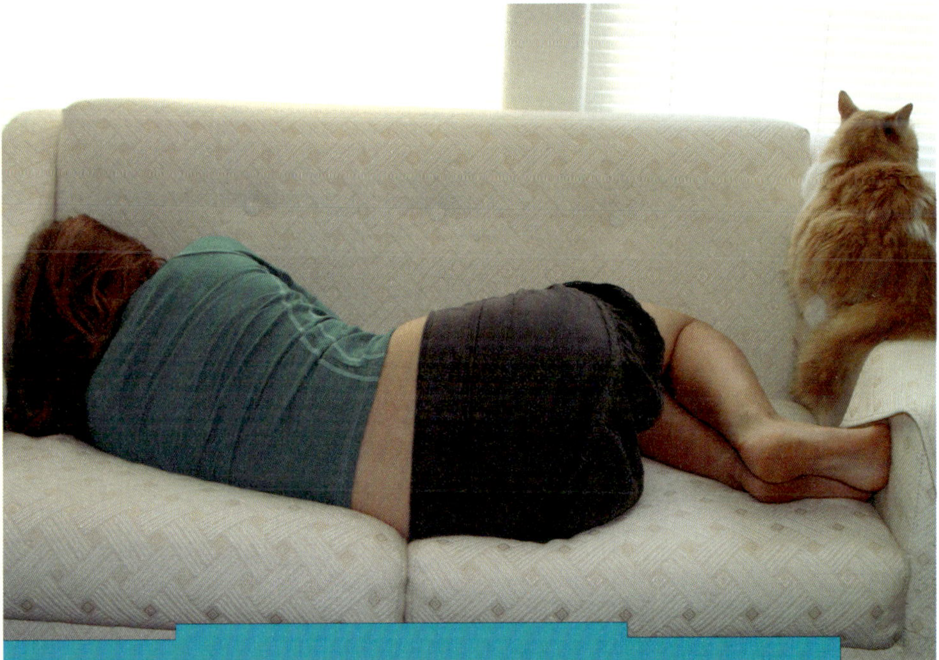

Even while sleeping, your body needs calories to fuel your heart, lungs, brain, and other organs and bodily systems.

billions of cells, whether you are running, sitting, lying down, or sleeping. And none of that work would get done without the fuel that comes from food. Your most important involuntary muscle, your heart, "works out" every minute of your life. Dozens of muscles contract and stretch so that you blink, yawn, swallow, and digest food—all without remembering to do any of these things. Your intentional motions—reaching, walking, talking, and smiling, to name just a few—require even more of the energy that comes from food.

Stored Energy

When the foods you eat provide less energy (which is measured in calories) than you use in a day, your body doesn't refuse to work. If it did, you'd stop breathing. Instead, it unlocks stored energy deposited throughout your body on the days when you ate more calories than you needed. The stored calories are now available from the fat and muscle tissue in your body.

Every body maintains a fat supply as its first source of stored energy. This is the most important reason why some amount of body fat is essential to good health. Your fat also helps maintain a healthy body temperature and cushions your bones. When a girl's or woman's fat supply falls far below healthy levels, her body stops producing estrogen. Menstruation (having your periods) can stop completely.

When there is neither food nor fat to meet the body's constant demands for energy, it still doesn't stop working, though it's tired and weak. To keep going, the body raids its muscle tissues for fuel, breaking them down and converting them back into nutrients to feed itself. Logically, this muscle loss is the last thing any athlete wants to have happen. Your muscle power is the athletic "motor" that you've trained and toned for top performance. Building up major muscle groups is a goal of most athletic training. Greater muscle mass improves your capacity to run, swim, leap, lift, stretch, and power a ball or a bicycle. Well-toned muscles also help deliver the bursts of speed that are critical in many sports. Without regular additions of energy-producing fuel to the body, this "motor" stops working. The smaller, weaker body won't go as far or as fast as it once did.

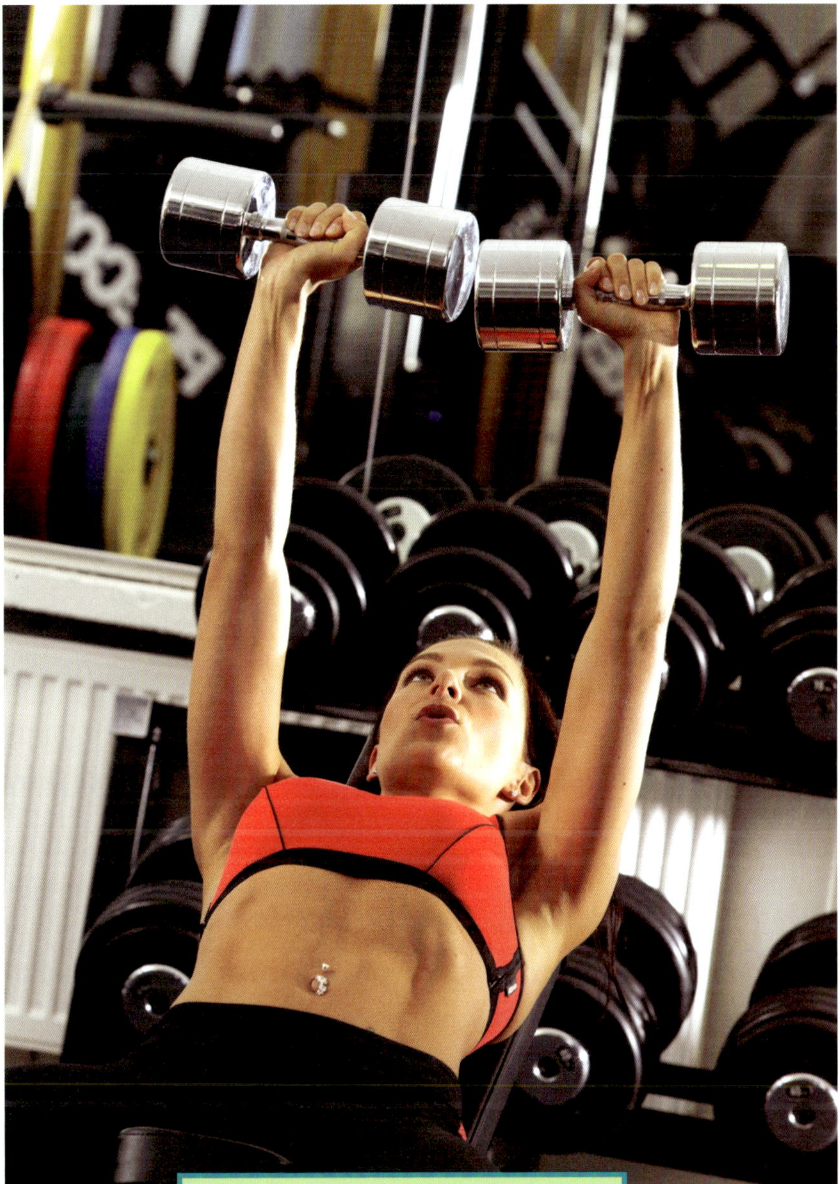

By not eating, athletes may destroy the very muscles that they work so hard to build.

Marathon runners eat big pasta dinners and other high-carbohydrate foods the day before a race. The body converts carbohydrates into energy at a slow, even pace, so they are a good source of energy for long races. Runners' energy needs are so big that without all this extra fuel, their bodies will consume all available body fat and sugars in less time than it takes to run twenty-six miles (41.8 kilometers). If a runner's muscle tissue is then "raided" to provide energy, he or she will get painful leg cramps and sudden weakness.

Vitamins and Minerals

Perhaps you don't run marathons, but you've had leg and foot cramps after some of your workouts? Maybe you've heard that vitamin supplements can help prevent cramps, so you take several different vitamin and mineral pills twice each day. Perhaps you think that vitamins can keep your strength up, or that they can take care of any gaps in your diet. Plus, they don't fill you up.

Even if you don't feel tired, vitamins do not supply energy or replace other nutrients. Only carbohydrates and fat can be readily used to supply energy. Vitamins and minerals are important to health because they help keep your arteries flexible and convert your food into muscle and other tissues. They also help maintain healthy hair and teeth. All the vitamins and minerals essential to good health occur naturally in some of the foods you eat. But they are not substances your body can convert into energy for sports. Vitamin pills and mixes cannot replace food.

Athletes frequently adopt training diets on their own or because their coach or trainer recommends a diet. There's nothing

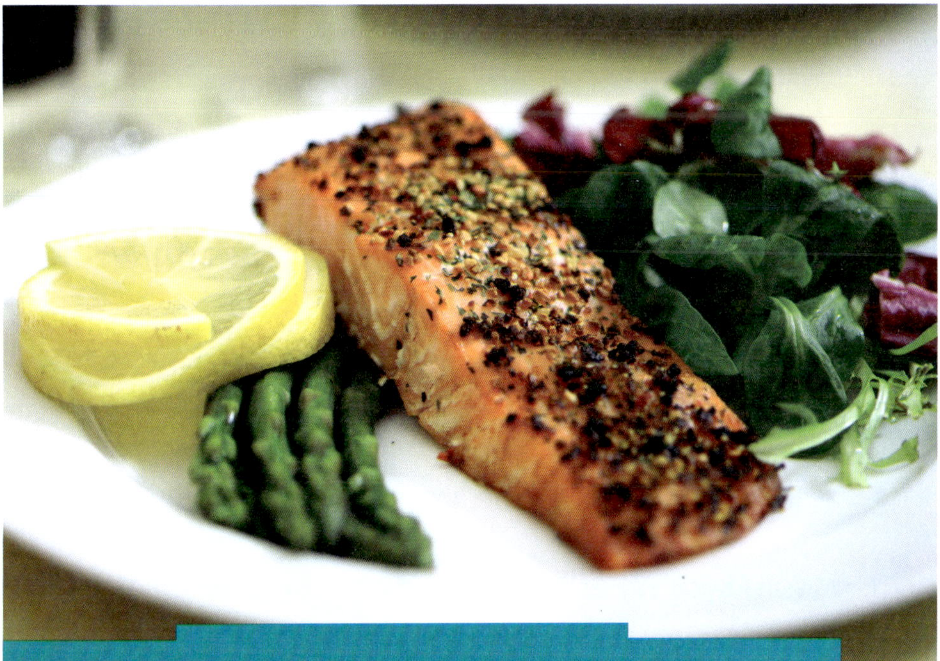

Simply eating is not necessarily enough to be healthy. Make sure each of your meals has the proper balance of protein, carbohydrates, and nutrients.

wrong with deciding to follow a plan. But it must be enough to sustain your extra physical effort. It should supply a proper balance of protein, carbohydrates, and fat.

To learn more about the relationship between eating, sports, and good health, ask your school nurse or librarian to recommend good resources, or check out the National Eating Disorders Association (NEDA) Web site at www.edap.org for additional information.

Myths and Facts

Myth **You are what you eat.** Fact ➜ Genetics matters more than diet, exercise, or any other single factor in the shape and size of your body.

Myth **Physically active people don't have to worry about how much they eat.** Fact ➜ When you exercise you use up more energy. Your body needs more fuel than less active people.

Myth **If I take vitamins, I don't have to worry about what I eat.** Fact ➜ Vitamins do not supply energy or replace other nutrients. Vitamin pills and mixes cannot replace food.

Myth **No one needs to worry about exercising too much.** Fact ➜ People who are addicted to exercise can have serious physical and emotional problems as a result of the disorder. They make exercise the most important thing in their lives. They have feelings of anxiety and guilt and they believe they are unattractive or out of control when they cannot exercise. Some even exercise when they are injured.

Myth

Wouldn't most athletes who perform well in their sport be excessive exercisers? Fact → Athletes should find a healthy balance of eating and exercise. According to a college sport nutritionist, an athlete who has an eating disorder cannot see food as fuel for his or her body but instead sees it as calories and fat. Initially, weight loss may improve an athlete's performance, but eventually compulsive exercise, restricting calories, or purging will affect the person's health negatively.

Myth

One of my coaches said that I was getting kind of big, so I think I need to go on a diet. Fact → Some coaches do not understand the effect their comments have on athletes. Most athletes will remember everything their coaches say and take it to heart. For many female athletes, dieting, excessive exercise, and low self-esteem begin when people such as their coaches focus on appearance, performance, and a lean body instead of on the whole person and her incentive and excitement for the sport.

Chapter three

WHAT LEADS TO EATING DISORDERS?

Some people don't believe that anorexia nervosa and bulimia nervosa are illnesses because many of the people who suffer from them strive to appear healthy, even "ideal." They are taught to practice self-discipline and to admire those who show it by getting good grades and becoming better athletes. They hold themselves to high standards and often juggle full schedules. You may measure your own dedication to your sport by noting all the things you give up—parties, television, vacations—to concentrate on it.

Self-Control

Eating disorders are illnesses, not weaknesses. Athletes and other strong, high-achieving people can develop them. (Young anorexia sufferers tend to have better

Though you should have enough self-control not to eat too much, that same self-control shouldn't drive you to starve yourself.

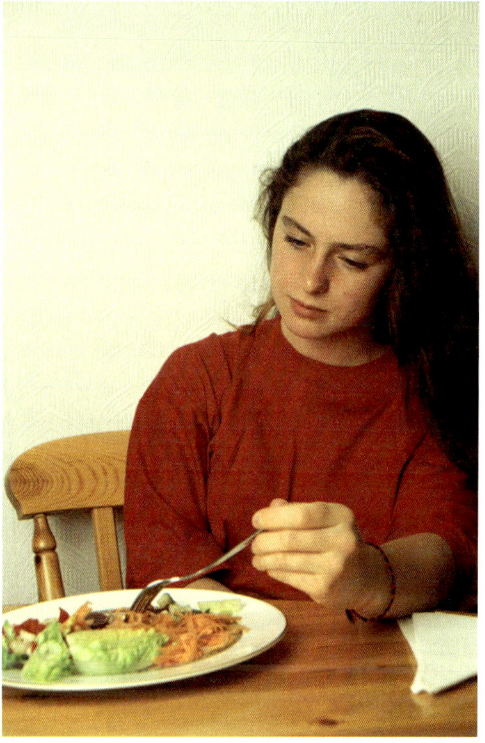

grades and higher ambitions, on average, than their peers who don't have an eating disorder.) They set personal goals that are admired by teammates, families, and friends. Young male athletes who develop eating disorders often begin by fasting or purging to meet personal or team goals for a specific sporting event or competition. They may be singled out by coaches and sportswriters as role models of dedication for less experienced athletes.

Self-control is a positive aspect of a person's character. Sadly, though, good self-control may actually make it easier for an athlete to develop an eating disorder. This is because he or she is willing to go hungry without complaining or "giving in" to food. In other words, the very things that make someone a good athlete—discipline, competitiveness, perfectionism—also contribute to eating disorders.

Being in Control

In your preteen and teen years, you'll probably become impatient to take control of some aspects of your life as you seek your own identity. Both food and sports can satisfy this need for control and independence. If you're putting in lots of time at the gym, rink, track, barre, or weight room to reach ever-higher performance levels, you're probably as tough on yourself as any coach. Meanwhile, your parents continue to expect you home at dinnertime, check your homework, or shop for clothes with you.

As control of your life is shifting—usually too slowly for you and too quickly for your parents—away from your parents and into your own hands, there are many areas of confusion, guesswork, and struggle. You may agree, for example, that you should have a curfew on school nights but feel that eight o'clock in the evening is too early. Or you may think it's fair that you do some housework, but not the chores your mom or dad want you to do. Many teens already control when and what they eat without drawing a lot of attention to themselves. They graze from the refrigerator when they please, have money for school lunches and fast food, and eat dinner earlier or later than the rest of the family in order to go to practices, games, and lessons.

Along with the need to assert control, many teens who develop eating disorders believe that to succeed in life they must change the way they look and reach an ideal set by others. Males and females with these disorders often believe that dieting or purging will help them attain beauty, popularity, or success, because their natural weight and natural eating habits aren't good enough. This attitude of low self-esteem is fed by the ideas

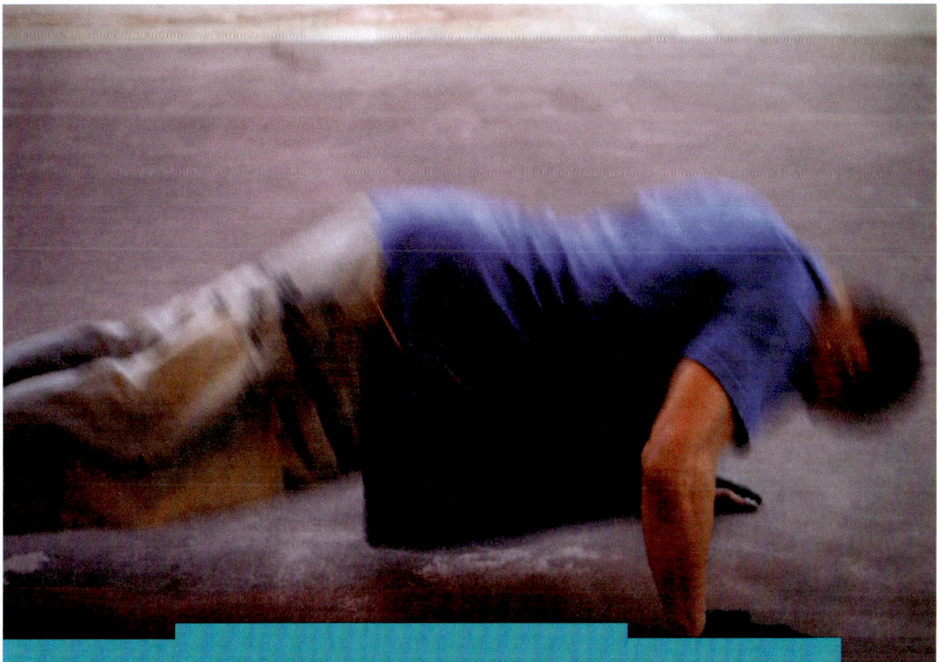

One symptom of eating disorders is overexercising. You should push yourself but not to the point where it jeopardizes your health.

that a thin, toned body is ideal and can be created by hard work. Even if you know this is wrong, the message is hard to ignore.

Most young women who stay in competitive sports show higher self-esteem and more self-discipline than classmates who don't commit to practicing and improving in sports. Even so, these young women may believe that their sport requires a very specific ideal body. In this situation, high self-esteem may not be enough to prevent eating disorders. For example, your love of dance is a positive emotion. But you also believe your pride in refusing dinner is positive. Ultimately, both make it easier for you not to eat.

Some athletes develop compulsive food and exercise rituals as a form of self-discipline. These rituals become the goals they can always achieve, unlike the games or races they can't win every time. If they get frustrated with a loss or a bad practice, skipping meals or doubling their workouts is their way of testing their willpower or punishing themselves for a "failure."

Other Factors That Can Lead to an Eating Disorder

There is no single cause for an eating disorder. Besides being linked to feelings of low self-esteem, eating disorders can be expressions of other concerns and issues in an individual's life. Many eating disorders originate from other pressures, such as those from family, friends, and society. (For example, American society places a great deal of importance on thinness, and various media, including TV, movies, and magazines, promote model-like thinness as being the "ideal" for beauty.) These other pressures can include physical, sexual, or emotional abuse; family problems; substance abuse; or changes or transitions in the person's life, such as going through puberty or moving to a new school or home.

How Do I Know If I Have a Problem?

A good character and a strong body cannot protect an athlete from developing an eating disorder. Are you wondering if you have eating habits that could hurt you? Answer these questions to help yourself decide. If you answer yes to these questions, please consider getting help.

Athletic performance is not the only trigger for eating disorders. Pressures, such as those at school, can also lead to excessive dieting.

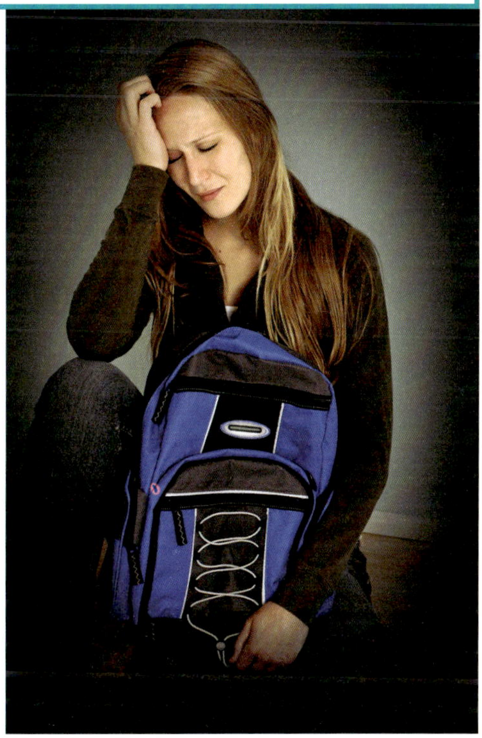

Is the habit a secret? Hiding your food choices, fasting, bingeing, or purging from others is a danger sign for eating disorders. If you think your eating patterns or weight-loss goals are too weird to explain to anyone, they probably are. If you're afraid to tell someone about them, why?

When someone offers nutrition advice or a food item, what happens? If a simple eating suggestion or the offer of a small treat makes you angry, you may be engaged in an emotional battle with that person. You may be struggling with that person about who is in control of your eating.

Do you buy, cook, or eat food just for yourself? Some athletes do this because they think no one else will understand or accept their food choices. Others are convinced that their special need to become faster, better, and stronger than the competition requires a diet too severe for "ordinary" people, especially the less athletic members of their own families.

If you feel that you're obsessing about food, by always having to control what and how much you eat, you may want to talk to a professional.

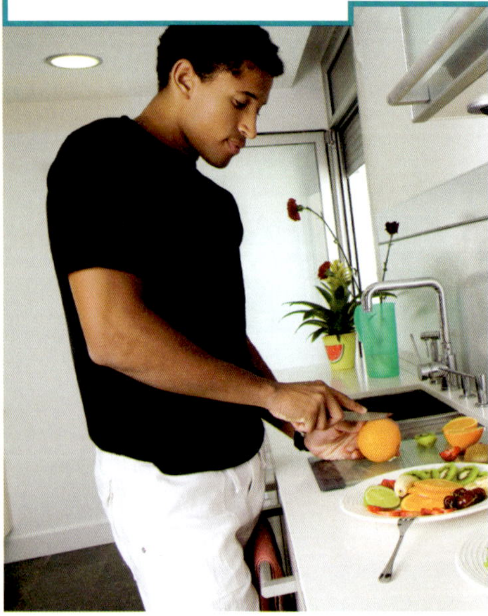

Are you afraid that if you stop your eating and exercise habits your life will be ruined? Believing that your whole future depends on what you eat is one of the signs of an eating disorder.

If you recognize that you might have an eating disorder, make an appointment with your doctor to enable him or her to make a diagnosis and then discuss your treatment plan with you and your family.

chapter four

WHAT ARE THE CONSEQUENCES OF EATING DISORDERS?

Anorexia and bulimia are dangerous illnesses that afflict hundreds of thousands of women and thousands of men every year. It is estimated that more than eleven million Americans suffer from eating disorders. According to H. W. Hoek and D. van Hoeken's article in *International Journal of Eating Disorders* (2003), 40 percent of the newly diagnosed cases of anorexia are females who are between the ages of fifteen and nineteen. Anorexia can even be fatal, killing six to eighteen of every one hundred people with the illness. Experts estimate that males make up from 5 to 15 percent of the people with anorexia or bulimia, and that about 35 percent of the people with binge eating disorder are male. (However, because not all people who have eating disorders go to health professionals for help, no one is really sure of the statistics.)

Learning the facts about eating disorders will help you realize that no athlete can get faster, stronger, and better at a sport because of an eating disorder.

What Is Anorexia Nervosa?

Anorexia nervosa, commonly called anorexia, is a deadly illness. Unlike the flu or a sexually transmitted disease (STD), anorexia isn't spread by bacteria or a virus. Instead, anorexia stems from your thoughts and emotions.

Currently, more than eight million Americans suffer from eating disorders. Ninety to 95 percent of those who suffer are female, and the number of males with eating disorders is increasing. There are many men and adolescent males who go undiagnosed either because of the lack of reporting the disorder or because of misdiagnoses.

Doctors are slowly beginning to better understand anorexia. There are now treatments that can help people who have anorexia gain self-esteem and get healthy.

About Anorexia Nervosa

You may have heard the term "anorexia" used before; maybe you talked about it in health class, read about it in a magazine, or heard someone talk about how actress Mary-Kate Olsen was being treated for it. Your mom may get upset if you don't want to finish your dinner and say, "Please eat! You haven't been eating enough food lately. You've lost some weight already. Are you still concerned about losing more weight? You aren't becoming ill are you?"

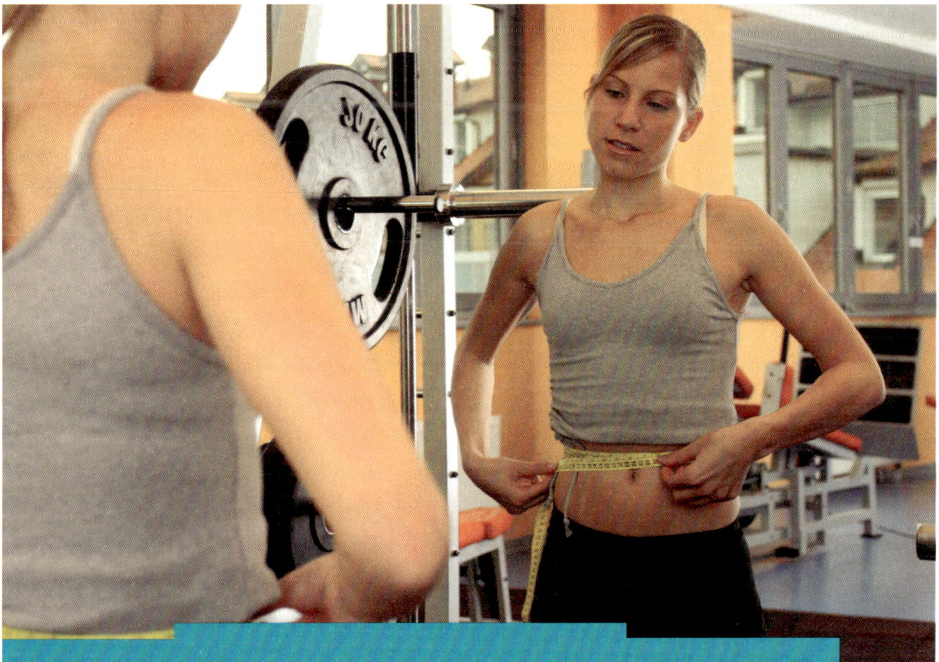

Just as obsessing about food may be a sign of an eating disorder, so is being overly concerned about your waistline.

Chances are, eating-related issues probably influence your life or that of a family member or friend right now. You or this person might already feel a few of the forces that cause an eating disorder to kick in: insecurity, peer pressure, or society's pressure to be thin.

The word "anorexia" literally means "loss of appetite." But anorexia is more like self-starvation—becoming so obsessed with losing weight and dieting that you ignore your body's hunger signals. Although people with anorexia are always hungry, they take pride in denying hunger, feeling more in control and independent. This belief has very dangerous consequences. If anorexia progresses far enough, you can lose massive amounts of body weight—enough to cause psychological problems, physical problems, and even death.

Anorexia nervosa is diagnosed in a person whose symptoms include the following:

- Weighs at least 15 percent less than the minimum average weight for his or her height, but has no physical illness that is causing the weight loss
- Has an intense fear of becoming fat
- "Sees" his or her body as overweight, despite being visibly underweight
- If a girl or woman of menstruating age has not had a period for at least three months.

What happens when a body is deprived of 15 percent or more of its minimum proper weight? In a matter of weeks or months, the person with anorexia experiences one, some, or all of the following physical problems:

Being frequently cold, even in summer or in a well-heated room. The body is burning up its essential fat stores to meet energy needs because there is no food in the system. As a result, the thin layer of subcutaneous (under-the-skin) fat is vanishing. This is the fat that helps you maintain normal body temperature.

Feeling light-headed and dizzy, possibly fainting. An anorexic athlete is depriving the heart, blood, brain, and other systems of vital supplies. Severe dieting means less blood is circulating through the body, causing lower blood pressure and

Anorexics, by definition, see themselves as fat when they are clearly dangerously thin.

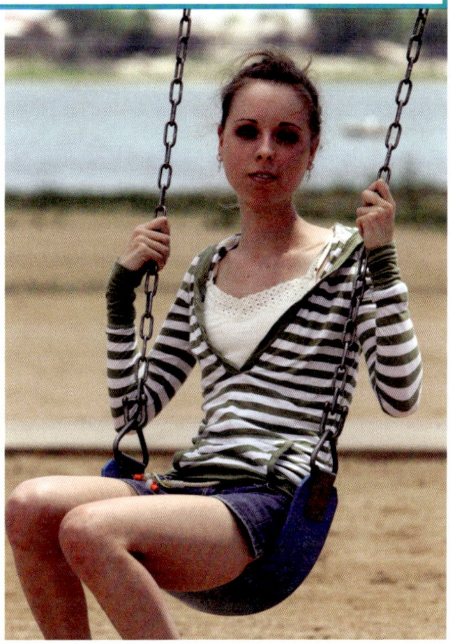

dizzy spells. Starvation also affects the heart muscle. Many anorexics develop a slow or irregular heartbeat.

Becoming more forgetful and having trouble concentrating. A person may feel irritable, unhappy, and pessimistic. These feelings are probably caused by the steady hunger and weakness that result from self-starvation. They can also be symptoms of depression, a dangerous emotional disorder that can occur whether or not an eating disorder is also present. If you have had these symptoms—changed sleeping patterns, feelings of hopelessness, inability to concentrate or remember things—for two weeks or more, speak to a trusted adult or a counselor at school.

Physical Consequences of Anorexia

Menstrual periods stop in a girl or woman who isn't pregnant when her body-fat stores are too low to support a healthy reproductive system. This condition is called amenorrhea. Anorexia is one cause of amenorrhea because of drastic weight loss. With treatment, she can begin eating adequately. When her weight and body fat climb back to minimum healthy levels, her periods will start again.

Osteoporosis, a condition in which bone mass is lost, is another danger signal. All sports, especially weight lifting and rowing, help to build bone mass, or bone density. Bone mass provides strength and support for all your weight-bearing activities, including walking, running, standing, or sitting. Bone building is a constant process requiring calcium and, in women, estrogen.

How can women athletes work out more than the average person but lose bone mass, when exercise increases bone mass? Health experts believe that when self-starvation becomes so severe that an anorexic woman stops getting her periods, she also produces less estrogen. Without enough estrogen to maintain and increase bone mass, her bones get weaker. They will shrink if the condition is not treated. If a young woman hasn't yet grown to her adult height, osteoporosis can stunt her growth.

Bone density is quickly lost but slowly restored. If you stayed in bed for just one week with the flu or a broken leg, you'd lose up to 1 percent of your bone mass, and you'd need four months on your feet to get it back. Weakened bones fracture more easily from the unavoidable stresses and impacts of sports: football tackles, gymnastic dismounts, and the pounding that runners absorb with every step.

The most serious complication of anorexia occurs when the body's digestive system simply shuts down and the person starves to death. This is rare, but so horrifying that many people

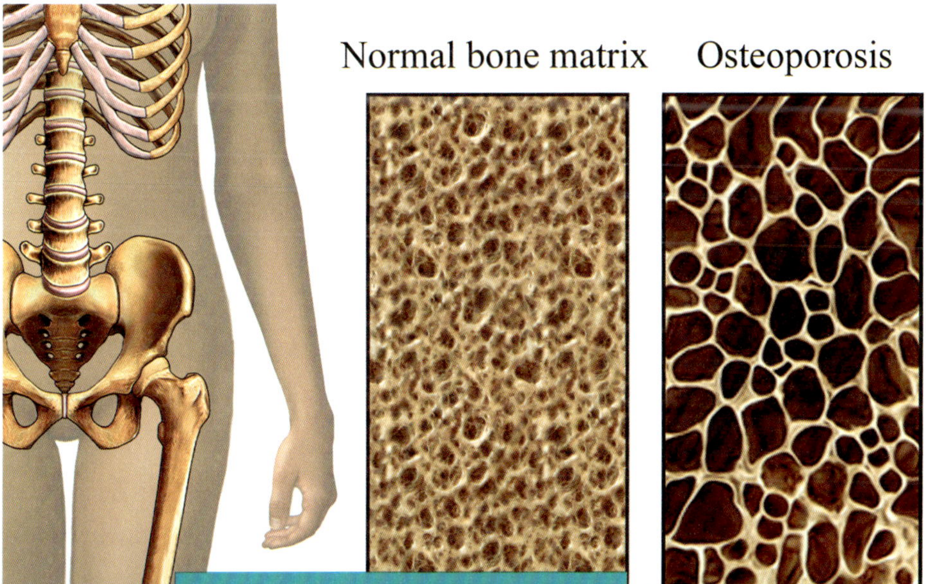

Osteoporosis is a serious medical condition, especially for women. As these images show, eating disorders can cause severe bone loss.

don't believe it can happen. The body's ability to process food, like muscle tone and memory, is something you have to use, or you'll lose it. People whose anorexia goes untreated can also suffer heart and kidney failure serious enough to kill them.

The Female Athlete Triad

Some athletes think that their good training habits and above-average strength will protect them from the bad effects of chronic undereating. This is not true. In fact, female athletes face an additional risk from untreated eating disorders. This risk is called the female athlete triad, after the three health problems that occur together in many women athletes: disordered eating, loss of menstrual periods, and loss of bone mass.

One of these conditions can signal that the body's essential nutrients and tissues are being "raided," usually by a combination of starvation and overexercising. When all three conditions appear at the same time, it is a health emergency. Experts say that as many as 30 percent of female athletes in sports such as gymnastics, long-distance running, and figure skating suffer from the female athlete triad, although the exact number is unknown. Studies concerning female college athletes have indicated that from 15 to 62 percent of female college athletes have eating disorder behaviors.

What Is Bulimia?

Bulimia nervosa is a type of eating disorder in which a person binges and purges. Bingeing means eating a large amount of food in a short period of time. Purging means getting rid of all the food by self-induced vomiting; abuse of laxatives, diet pills, and/or diuretics; excessive exercise; or fasting.

Bingeing can mean eating a lot of calories—as many as five thousand or more at a time. People with bulimia can binge once in a while, or twenty times each day or more. Then they will purge to rid their bodies of the extra calories. They may purge even after eating small amounts of food.

There are two types of bulimia: purging and non-purging. People with the purging type get rid of food in different ways.

Some people purge by self-induced vomiting. Others use drugs, such as diuretics (pills that increase urination), diet pills, laxatives (usually mild drugs that induce bowel movements), or enemas (liquids injected into the anus for cleansing the bowels) to clear the digestive tract. Both bingeing and purging can be experienced as intense, overwhelming urges that become uncontrollable. People with the non-purging type of bulimia exercise compulsively to get rid of the extra food they've eaten or rely on fasting.

Symptoms of Bulimia

It can be difficult to tell if a person has an eating disorder. Bulimia is especially tough to diagnose because the problem is often hidden.

Many people struggle with their relationship to food. We are taught from an early age to feel anxious and guilty around food, to worry about our weight, and to fear fat. People who are in the early stages of bulimia (or another eating disorder) may be overly concerned with their weight, but that isn't out of the ordinary in our culture.

People with bulimia are also not always really skinny, as you might think they would be. They can be of normal weight, or even overweight.

Warning Signs of Bulimia

Even though people with bulimia may not look different from anyone else, there are warning signs of the condition. People with the disorder may use extreme methods to lose weight, and they may act different from how they used to act. It's important to recognize these warning signs so that you can help yourself or help someone else who is struggling with bulimia. An eating disorder left untreated can be life threatening.

People with bulimia may do one or more of these things:

- Believe that they would be happier and more successful if they were thinner
- Have severe mood swings
- Overeat in response to stress or other uncomfortable feelings
- Alternate between strict dieting and overeating
- Go to the bathroom a lot to throw up after eating
- Exercise all the time
- Buy or steal large amounts of food
- Buy products like laxatives or syrup of ipecac (used to induce vomiting)

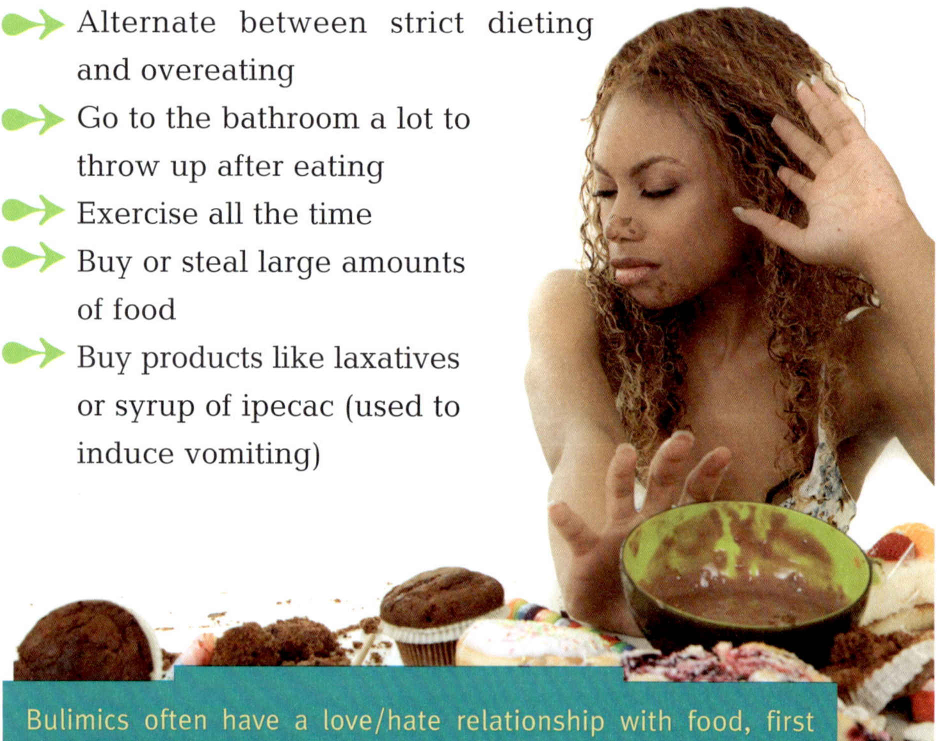

Bulimics often have a love/hate relationship with food, first bingeing on as much as they can, then purging it through vomiting or other means.

- Have cuts or marks on their knuckles and fingertips from using their fingers to induce vomiting
- Show other types of impulsive behavior, such as abusing drugs, going on shopping sprees, and/or shoplifting.

Diagnosing Bulimia Nervosa

A person who suffers from this binge-and-purge disorder faces damaging his or her health. Bulimia nervosa is diagnosed in a person who:

- Overeats in repeated food "binges" for three months or more and feels that he or she cannot stop eating during a binge
- Compensates for binges and tries to avoid gaining weight by vomiting, taking laxatives or other diet drugs, fasting, or excessive exercise
- Ties his or her self-esteem to appearance and weight.

Eating disorder experts believe that someone with bulimia can't tell the difference between the sensation of hunger and such seemingly overwhelming emotional sensations as anxiety, embarrassment, and fear. In other words, he or she "feels" nervousness about a final exam, a big swim meet, or a move to a new town as an urge to eat.

A person with bulimia shops or raids the refrigerator for huge amounts of food, much of it snack food or sweets, which is eaten quickly and usually alone. This person then gets the food out of the system after eating by vomiting. People with bulimia learn to provoke vomiting, usually by sticking their fingers far down

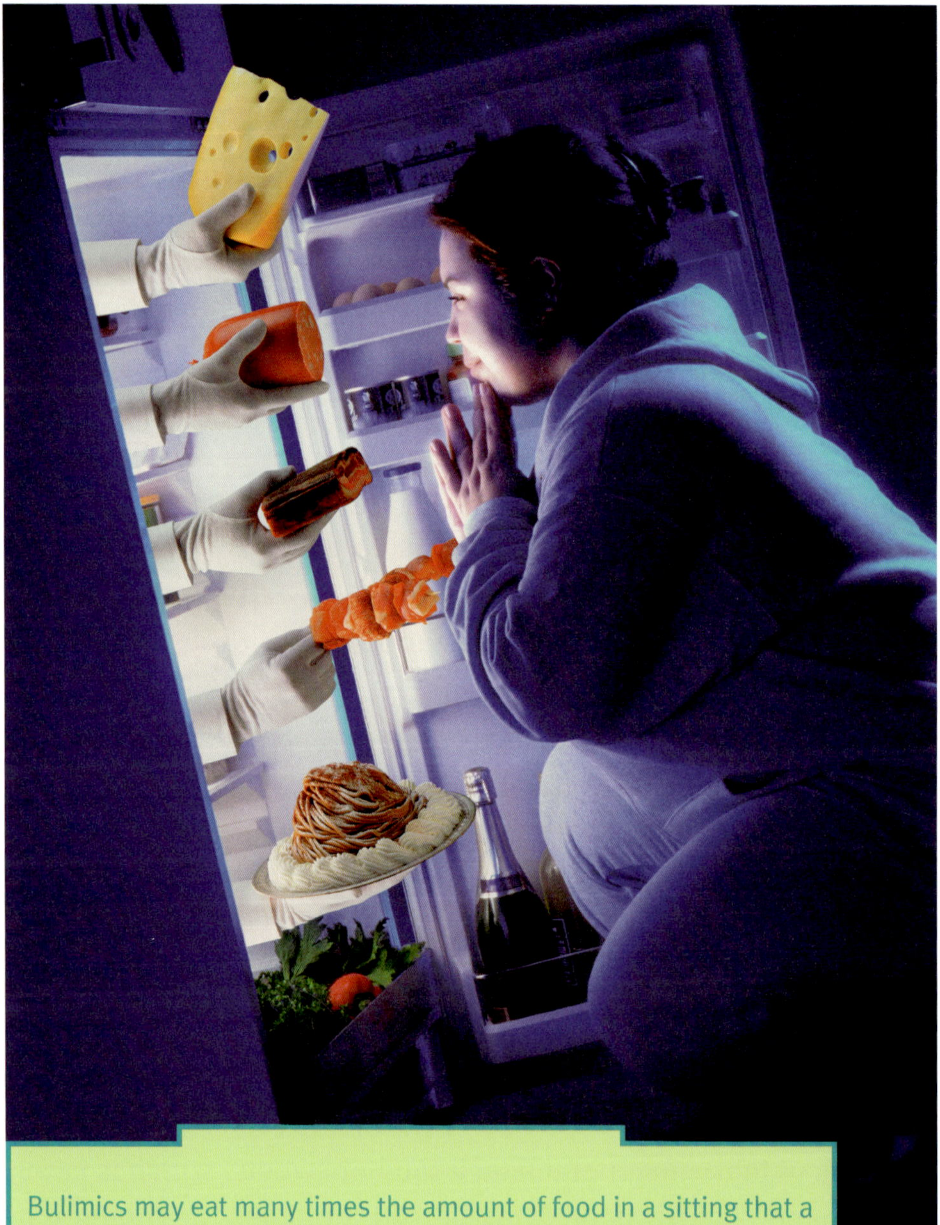

Bulimics may eat many times the amount of food in a sitting that a non-bulimic eats in an entire day, only to purge it soon afterward.

their throats. Certain medical research has found that the purge itself releases serotonin, a brain chemical that influences mood, and could actually make the purge feel good. Some people with bulimia have said that the feeling of peace, relief, and emptiness they feel during a purge is just as pleasurable as the binge itself.

People suffering from bulimia also may get rid of the food they consume during binges by taking over-the-counter drugs such as laxatives or diuretics that rush the food through their systems. Athletes may think there's a short-term advantage for losing the "extra baggage" in their stomachs before qualifying weigh-ins or short, intense events like the fifty-yard dash, hurdles, swimming relays, and wrestling matches.

Physical Consequences of Bulimia

By upsetting normal digestive processes, bulimia causes many health problems. A bulimic person's disorder and its complications often go unnoticed because the binges are kept secret. Unlike the person with anorexia who is noticeably "too skinny," the person with bulimia is less likely to be seriously underweight or to stop eating regular meals.

It can be difficult to tell if an individual has bulimia because the disorder is frequently hidden and the person may not look different from anyone else. The most obvious symptoms are the cuts or marks on the person's knuckles and fingertips from using the fingers to induce vomiting, and bloodshot eyes that result after a purge. Other symptoms include dry skin, brittle nails, or bleeding gums caused by the lack of vitamins and minerals in the body. Purging rituals get food out of the body before its

Constant vomiting can cause serious damage to the throat, mouth, and teeth and may require extensive and expensive dental work.

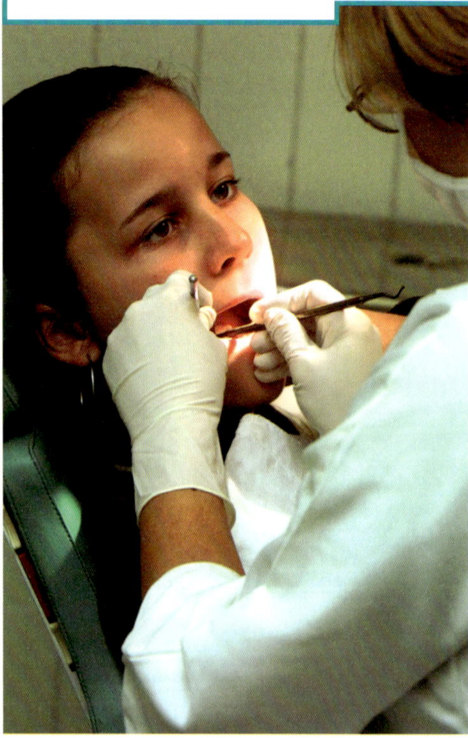

nutrients can be absorbed. Without these nutrients, the body can suffer from malnutrition even if that person is not too thin and eats regular meals at other times. In addition to tiredness, skin problems, gum problems, and eyesight that is weak, vitamin and mineral deficiencies can cause serious unseen harm to the bulimic person's heart, kidneys, and bones.

The teeth develop cavities or raggedy edges, and the gums may be swollen and tender. This happens because vomiting brings stomach acids up to the mouth. These acids, strong enough to break down foods, are also strong enough to wear away tooth enamel and the softer tissues of the mouth. If a person vomits frequently, he or she is likely to develop tooth decay and gum disease.

A bulimic person will have stomach pains. Vomiting is a violent reflex that batters the esophagus and stomach lining. The damage is invisible but so serious that it can be painful for a person to swallow anything, even water. A person may also have frequent cramps and indigestion. If someone purges frequently with laxatives, he or she may become dependent on them for normal bowel movements.

If you think you may suffer from an eating disorder, it's extremely important to get help. Consider speaking with someone you trust, such as a parent, a friend, or a counselor. Recovery is a long process, but with help, you can get better.

Chapter five

DO I HAVE AN EATING DISORDER?

Anorexia and bulimia are serious illnesses that must be diagnosed by a doctor, and people who suffer from them need treatment to get better. Athletes who experiment with starving, bingeing, and purging can get hurt, even if they don't have an eating disorder. Their experiments, called disordered eating behaviors, are risky because they can become habits, then uncontrollable urges. Even a single episode, if it is very extreme, can make an athlete so tired, thirsty, or dizzy that he or she gets injured or sick. An athlete who can honestly say "I don't have an eating disorder" may still have a troubled relationship with food and body size.

Males and Eating Disorders

Most male athletes never try a slow, gradual weight-loss program because they don't need to lose weight. But they

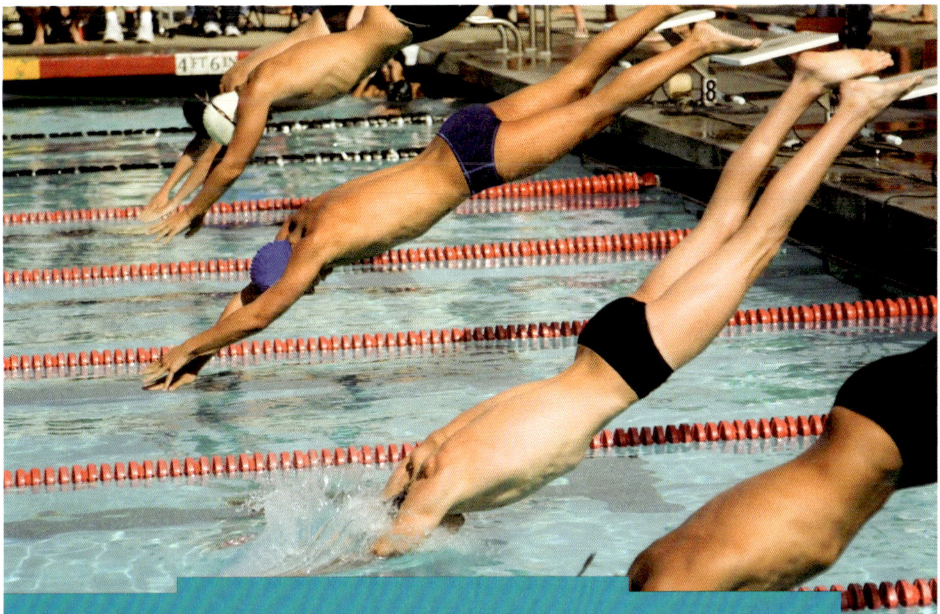

Weight-sensitive sports, such as track, wrestling, horse racing, and swimming, often lead male participants to develop eating disorders.

may try to lose or gain pounds quickly for a competitive edge in a big game or meet. Afterward, they'll return to pregame form in a day or two. Despite this "game day" approach to disordered eating, some males develop anorexia or bulimia. Experts estimate that about one million males, not all of them athletes, will develop an eating disorder at some time. This is only about one-tenth the number of women who will develop an eating disorder.

In sports where weight or body-fat percentage is closely monitored—such as wrestling, swimming, and track—male athletes are more likely to use over-the-counter drugs to drop a few pounds for a day. Boys and men who are willing to manipulate their weight and shape to reach athletic goals are also more likely to abuse drugs such as anabolic steroids, which can speed up the growth of muscle tissue, or so-called fat-burning drugs and food supplements.

Men who suffer from eating disorders will have different role models, performance goals, and body ideals than women, but their physical symptoms (except for amenorrhea), distorted perceptions, and fear of fat are the same. The high-risk sports for men, like those for women, are the ones where appearance is a big factor in success: bodybuilding, diving, figure skating, and gymnastics.

"I Don't Have an Eating Disorder Because . . ."

There are many ways to finish the sentence "I don't have an eating disorder because . . . " Perhaps you've heard some of them yourself: ". . . guys can't get eating disorders," or ". . . I never throw up," or ". . . I eat three meals a day," or ". . . I'm never very hungry." Athletes have many different reasons for saying they don't have an eating disorder. Some of them may fear getting kicked off the team. Others will be embarrassed because they think eating disorders are personality flaws or that no one in their sport ever gets an eating disorder. While there are real differences between them, disordered eating can certainly lead to a serious eating disorder. Recognizing the signs and symptoms of disordered eating early can help prevent the development of eating disorders.

Helping a Friend

If you're worried that a friend may have an eating disorder, what can you do? First, remember that eating disorders are illnesses, and you're not a doctor. You can't cure someone's harmful eating behaviors. Second, you want your friend to feel better and eat better, but you can't make her or him do anything. Here are some dos and don'ts for raising your concerns:

- **DO** plan this conversation for a quiet time and place. Creating privacy for a serious talk about personal issues shows your respect, and your friend won't feel trapped.
- **DO** think about what you will say in advance. Have a plan to end the talk if you begin arguing with each other.
- **DO** ask another person who knows your friend and shares your concern to do this with you.
- **DO** have an eating disorders hotline number, brochure, or book with you. When the conversation ends, offer to leave it with your friend.
- **DON'T** make demands like "Stop doing this to yourself" or "Start eating like everyone else." Eating disorders are illnesses. A person can't stop anorexia or bulimia without treatment any more than he or she can stop an allergy or a sprained ankle.
- **DON'T** tell your friend, "You're not yourself anymore" or "People are talking about you." Even if it's true, it won't help. The purpose of your talk is to help! Your friend will stop listening, and your message will be lost.

What Is an Eating Disorder?

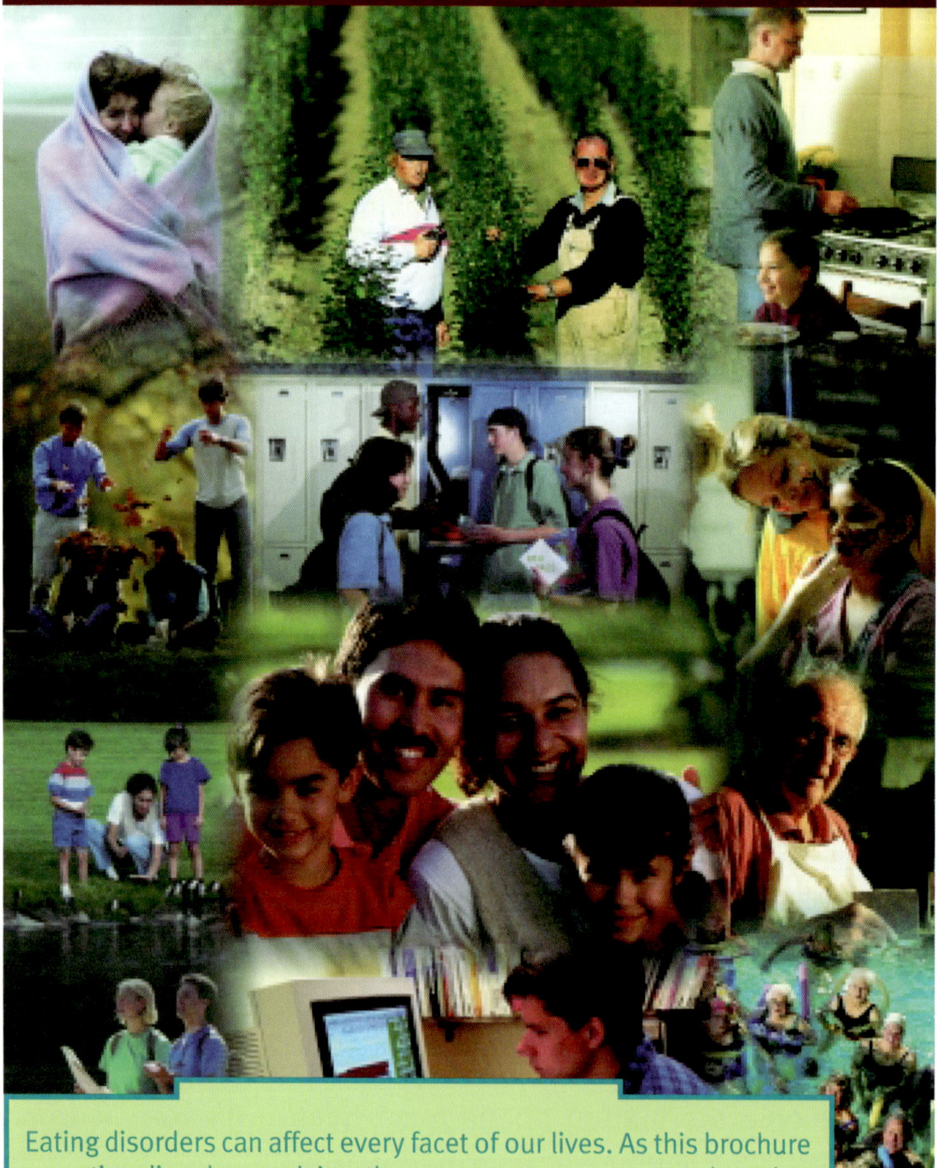

Eating disorders can affect every facet of our lives. As this brochure on eating disorders explains, there are ways to prevent and combat the disease.

- **DON'T** bargain: "If you'll stop dieting, I'll stop biting my nails," or "If you don't stop, I can't be your friend." Just state your concern and your wish for your friend to seek help. If he or she refuses, say, "I may talk to you about this another day if I think you're not getting better. I care about you even if you don't agree with what I'm saying."
- **DON'T** wait for a right time to talk if your friend is already physically ill or has signs of severe depression. Instead, tell a responsible adult right away, and ask him or her to help.

Even when eating disorders are identified, treatment can take months or years. Doctors, therapists, supportive family, and teammates can help athletes learn new ways of thinking and feeling about how they eat, why they perform, and what it means to be healthy.

Your body needs to see you through many more years of life. You can't know today what physical stresses will challenge you in the future, but you'll certainly meet many different ones. Your most rewarding feat may be finishing a marathon, competing in a championship event, having a family, campaigning door-to-door for public office, or lugging a cello to concert dates. Your healthy body and strong self-image are two of the most important allies you'll ever have, and you are the only person who can keep them both on your side.

Ten Great Questions to Ask a Doctor

1. What is an appropriate weight for my height?

2. How can I lose weight safely?

3. How much exercise is recommended for teens to maintain a healthy body?

4. If I exercise regularly, do I still need to pay attention to good nutrition?

5. What causes exercise addiction?

6. Does exercise addiction cause other health problems?

7. What are the treatments for eating disorders/exercise addiction?

8 How will I know if I am improving?

9 How long does it take to be cured of my eating disorder/exercise addiction?

10 Are there different degrees of eating disorders/exercise addiction?

Glossary

addiction An obsessive/compulsive need for and use of a substance or behavior.

amenorrhea The disappearance of menstrual periods in women who are not pregnant.

body image The way you perceive your body and how you think others perceive your body.

carbohydrate An essential nutrient found in sugars, starches, grains, beans, fruits, and vegetables.

dehydration When the body loses water and other fluids it needs.

deprivation The act of withholding something.

diuretic A substance that speeds water's removal from the body, usually by urination.

esophagus The throat.

estrogen A female hormone.

fasting To stop eating food for a period of time.

genetic Relating to how people inherit traits and appearances from their parents.

indigestion Inability to digest food.

laxative A substance that brings on a bowel movement.

malnutrition Bad nutrition.

minerals Elements found in food that help to keep the body healthy and normal.

nutrient Something that provides nourishment.

nutrition How the body processes food.

osteoporosis A disease characterized by a decrease in bone mass, causing bones to weaken and break easily.

perfectionism The belief that anything that isn't perfect is not acceptable.

protein An essential part of our body's cells and a nutrient found in meat, milk, fish, and poultry.

self-discipline Giving oneself strict rules to follow in order to improve.

starvation Extreme hunger; to perish from lack of food.

For More Information

Alliance for Eating Disorders Awareness
P.O. Box 13155
North Palm Beach, FL 33408-3155
(866) 662-1235
Web site: http://www.eatingdisorderinfo.org

This organization tries to establish easily accessible programs in the United States that allow children and young adults the opportunity to learn about eating disorders and the positive effects of a healthy body image. Its aim is to disseminate educational information to the public about the warning signs, dangers, and consequences of anorexia, bulimia, and other related disorders, including exercise addiction.

American Dietetic Association
120 South Riverside Plaza, Suite 208
Chicago, IL 60606-6995
(800) 877-1600
Web site: http://www.eatright.org

This organization offers food and nutrition information for maintaining a healthy diet.

Anorexia Nervosa and Related Eating Disorders, Inc. (ANRED)
P.O. Box 5102
Eugene, OR 97405
(503) 344-1144
Web site: http://www.anred.com

ANRED provides information about food and weight disorders, including those that affect athletes. It offers suggestions for self-help and important information about recovery and prevention of these disorders.

Food and Nutrition Information Center (FNIC)
Agricultural Research Service, USDA
National Agricultural Library, Room 105
10301 Baltimore Avenue
Beltsville, MD 20705-2351
(301) 504-5719
Web site: http://www.nal.usda.gov/fnic

The FNIC staff is made up of nutrition professionals, most of whom are registered dieticians, who provide a wealth of knowledge about food and nutrition. The Web site contains more than two thousand links to reliable nutrition information.

Helping to End Eating Disorders (HEED)
191 Sweet Hollow Road
Old Bethpage, NY 11804
(516) 694-1054

Web site: http://www.helpingendeatingdisorders.org

HEED can help young people and their families deal with eating disorders. They refer the public to individuals or groups who offer many different kinds of therapy.

National Association of Anorexia Nervosa and Associated Disorders (ANAD)
P.O. Box 7
Highland Park, IL 60035
(847) 831-3438
Web site: http://www.anad.org

This organization offers information about services and programs in the prevention and treatment of eating disorders, and support for people who are seeking help.

National Eating Disorders Association (NEDA)
603 Stewart Street, Suite 803
Seattle, WA 98101
(800) 931-2237
Web site: http://www.edap.org

A not-for-profit organization, NEDA offers education, treatment, prevention, and research information regarding eating disorders.

National Institute of Mental Health (NIMH)
National Institutes of Health
U.S. Department of Health and Human Services
NIMH Public Information and Communications Branch
6001 Executive Boulevard, Room 8184, MSC 9663
Bethesda, MD 20892-9663

(301) 443-4513 or (866) 615-6464

Web site: http://www.nimh.nih.gov

The U.S. government's agency for research on mental and behavioral disorders. It provides information on eating disorders and the various clinical studies that are in progress or have been completed, and other medical and educational services that are available to the public.

Obsessive Compulsive Foundation

676 State Street

New Haven, CT 06511

(203) 401-2070

Web site: http://www.ocfoundation.org

This organization offers information on obsessive-compulsive disorder and support groups.

Web Sites

Due to the changing nature of Internet links, Rosen Publishing has developed an online list of Web sites related to the subject of this book. This site is updated regularly. Please use this link to access the list:

http://www.rosenlinks.com/faq/aaed

For Further Reading

Cirrone, Dorian. *Dancing in Red Shoes Will Kill You*. New York, NY: HarperCollins, 2005.

Kingsbury, Kathleen-Burns, and Mary Ellen Williams. *Weight Wisdom*. New York, NY: Taylor and Francis, 2003.

Kittleson, Mark J., ed. *The Truth About Eating Disorders*. New York, NY: Facts on File, 2005.

Lawton, Sandra Augustyn, ed. *Eating Disorders Information for Teens: Health Tips About Anorexia, Bulimia, Binge Eating, and Other Eating Disorders*. Detroit. MI: Omnigraphics, 2005.

Litt, Ann. *Fuel for Young Athletes: Essential Foods and Fluids for Future Champions*. Champaign, IL: Human Kinetics, 2004.

Orr, Tamra B. *When the Mirror Lies: Anorexia, Bulimia, and Other Eating Disorders*. New York, NY: Franklin Watts, 2006.

Otis, Carol L., and Roger Goldingay. *The Athletic Woman's Survival Guide: How to Win the Battle Against Eating Disorders, Amenorrhea, and Osteoporosis*. Champaign, IL: Human Kinetics, 2000.

Prussin, Rebecca, Philip D. Harvey, and Theresay Foy Digeronimo. *Hooked on Exercise: How to Understand and Manage Exercise Addiction*. New York, NY: Fireside Parkside, 1992.

Schlosser, Eric. *Chew on This: Everything You Don't Want to Know About Fast Food*. Boston, MA: Houghton Mifflin, 2006.

Sherman, Roberta Trattner, and Ron A. Thompson. *Helping Athletes with Eating Disorders*. Champaign, IL: Human Kinetics Publishers, 1993.

Sparks, Beatrice. *Kim: Empty Inside*. New York, NY: Avon, 2002.

Walsh, B. Timothy, and V. L. Cameron. *If Your Adolescent Has an Eating Disorder*. New York, NY: Oxford University Press, 2005.

Whytock, Cherry. *My Cup Runneth Over: The Life of Angelica Cookson Potts*. New York, NY: Simon and Schuster, 2003.

Index

About the Author

Barbara Zahensky has written articles on several eating disorders for Rosen's Teen Health & Wellness database. She lives in Yorktown, New York.

Photo Credits

Cover © www.istockphoto.com/Forest Woodward; pp. 5, 35 © AP Images; p. 7 © Bob Daemmrich/The Image Works; p. 9 © Elsa/Getty Images; p. 11 © Chabruken/The Image Bank/Getty Images; p. 13 © www.istockphoto.com/james boulette; p. 16 © Jed Jacobsohn/Getty Images; p. 17 © www.istockphoto.com/Paige Falk; pp. 19, 29 © Shutterstock.com; p. 21 © www.istockphoto.com/Branislav Senic; p. 25 © Herc Robinson/Bubbles Photolibrary/Alamy; p. 27 © www.istockphoto.com/Hélène Vallée; p. 30 © www.istockphoto.com/Alex Brosa; p. 33 © www.istockphoto.com/Tomaz Levstek; p. 37 Illustration © 2007 Nucleus Medical Art, All rights reserved. www.nucleusinc.com; p. 40 © www.istockphoto.com/Simone van den Berg; p. 42 © Alberto Incrocci/The Image Bank/Getty Images; p. 44 © www.istockphoto.com/Millanovic; p. 47 © www.istockphoto.com/Chad McDermott.

Designer: Evelyn Horovicz; Editor: Nicholas Croce;
Photo Researcher: Amy Feinberg